Pale

Diet Cookbook

Reduce Inflammation, Feel Vibrant and Burn Fat Quickly With Healthy Pegan Recipes.

Kaylin Wiza

The following Book is reproduced below with the goal of providing information that is as accurate and reliable as possible. Regardless, purchasing this Book can be seen as consent to the fact that both the publisher and the author of this book are in no way experts on the topics discussed within and that any recommendations or suggestions that are made herein are for entertainment purposes only. Professionals should be consulted as needed prior to undertaking any of the action endorsed herein.

This declaration is deemed fair and valid by both the American Bar Association and the Committee of Publishers Association and is legally binding throughout the United States.

Additionally, the information in the following pages is intended only for informational purposes and should thus be thought of as universal. As befitting its nature, it is presented without assurance regarding its prolonged validity or interim quality. Trademarks that are mentioned are done without written consent and can in no way be considered an endorsement from the trademark holder.

Table of Contents

BREAKFAST

1. Egg White Scramble with Cherry Tomatoes & Spinach

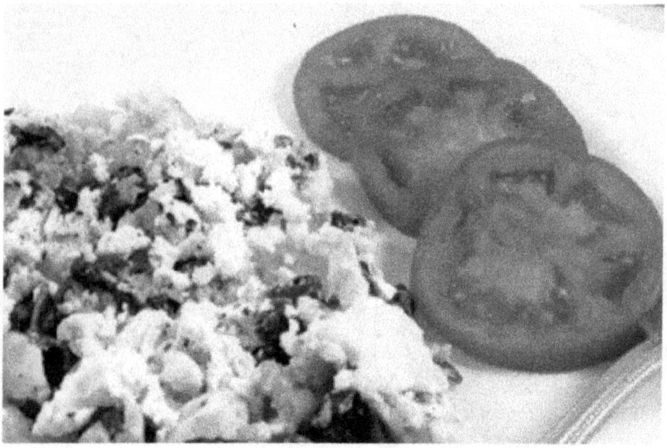

Preparation Time: 5 minutes

Cooking Time: 8-10 minutes

Servings: 4

INGREDIENTS:

- 1 tbsp. Olive oil
- 1 whole Egg
- 10 Egg whites
- ¼ tsp. Black pepper
- ½ tsp. Salt

- 1 garlic clove, minced
- 2 cups cherry tomatoes, halved
- 2 cups packed fresh baby spinach
- ½ cup Light cream or Half & Half
- ¼ cup finely grated parmesan cheese

DIRECTIONS:

1. Whisk the eggs, pepper, salt, and milk. Prepare a skillet using the med-high temperature setting. Toss in the garlic when the pan is hot to sauté for approximately 30 seconds.
2. Pour in the tomatoes and spinach and continue to sauté it for one additional minute. The tomatoes should be softened, and the spinach wilted.
3. Add the egg mixture into the pan using the medium heat setting. Fold the egg gently as it cooks for about two to three minutes. Remove from the burner, and sprinkle with a sprinkle of cheese.

NUTRITION: Calories 142 Protein: 15g Fat: 2g Carbs 4g

2. Greek Yogurt with Fresh Berries, Honey and Nuts

Preparation time: 5 minutes

Cooking time: 0 minutes

Servings: 1

INGREDIENTS:

- 6 oz. nonfat plain Greek yogurt
- 1/2 cup fresh berries of your choice
- 1 tbsp .25 oz crushed walnuts
- 1 tbsp honey

DIRECTIONS:

1. In a jar with a lid, add the yogurt. Top with berries and a drizzle of honey. Top with the lid and store in the fridge for 2-3 days.

NUTRITION: Calories: 250 Carbs: 35 Fat: 4g Protein: 19g

3. Mediterranean Egg Muffins with Ham

Preparation time: 15 minutes

Cooking time: 15 minutes

Servings: 6

INGREDIENTS:

- 9 Slices of thin cut deli ham
- 1/2 cup canned roasted red pepper, sliced + additional for garnish
- 1/3 cup fresh spinach, minced
- 1/4 cup feta cheese, crumbled
- 5 large eggs
- Pinch of salt
- Pinch of pepper
- 1 1/2 tbsp Pesto sauce
- Fresh basil for garnish

DIRECTIONS:

1. Preheat oven to 400 degrees F. Spray a muffin tin with cooking spray, generously. Line each of the muffin tin with 1 ½ pieces of ham - making sure there aren't any holes for the egg mixture come out.

2. Place some of the roasted red pepper in the bottom of each muffin tin. Place 1 tbsp of minced spinach on top of each red pepper. Top the pepper and spinach off with a large 1/2 tbsp of crumbled feta cheese.
3. In a medium bowl, whisk together the eggs salt and pepper, divide the egg mixture evenly among the 6 muffin tins.
4. Bake for 15 to 17 minutes until the eggs are puffy and set. Remove each cup from the muffin tin. Allow to cool completely
5. Distribute the muffins among the containers, store in the fridge for 2 - 3days or in the freezer for 3 months.

NUTRITION: Calories: 109 Carbs: 2g Fat: 6g Protein: 9g

4. Quinoa Bake with Banana

Preparation time: 15 minutes

Cooking time: 1 hour & 10 minutes

Servings: 8

INGREDIENTS:

- 3 cups medium over-ripe Bananas, mashed
- 1/4 cup molasses
- 1/4 cup pure maple syrup
- 1 tbsp cinnamon
- 2 tsp raw vanilla extract
- 1 tsp ground ginger
- 1 tsp ground cloves
- 1/2 tsp ground allspice
- 1/2 tsp salt
- 1 cup quinoa, uncooked
- 2 1/2 cups unsweetened vanilla almond milk
- 1/4 cup slivered almonds

DIRECTIONS:

1. In the bottom of a 2 1/2-3-quart casserole dish, mix together the mashed banana, maple syrup, cinnamon, vanilla extract, ginger, cloves, allspice, molasses, and salt until well mixed.

2. Add in the quinoa, stir until the quinoa is evenly in the banana mixture. Whisk in the almond milk, mix until well combined, cover and refrigerate overnight or bake immediately.
3. Heat oven to 350 degrees F. Whisk the quinoa mixture making sure it doesn't settle to the bottom.
4. Cover the pan with tinfoil and bake until the liquid is absorbed, and the top of the quinoa is set, about 1 hour to 1 hour and 15 minutes.
5. Turn the oven to high broil, uncover the pan, sprinkle with sliced almonds, and lightly press them into the quinoa.
6. Broil until the almonds just turn golden brown, about 2-4 minutes, watching closely, as they burn quickly. Allow to cool for 10 minutes then slice the quinoa bake
7. Distribute the quinoa bake among the containers, store in the fridge for 3-4 days.

NUTRITION: Calories: 213 Carbs: 41g Fat: 4g Protein: 5g

5. Italian Breakfast Sausage with Baby Potatoes and Vegetables

Preparation time: 15 minutes

Cooking time: 30 minutes

Servings: 4

INGREDIENTS:

- 1 lb. sweet Italian sausage links, sliced on the bias (diagonal)
- 2 cups baby potatoes, halved
- 2 cups broccoli florets
- 1 cup onions cut to 1-inch chunks
- 2 cups small mushrooms -half or quarter the large ones for uniform size
- 1 cup baby carrots
- 2 tbsp olive oil
- 1/2 tsp garlic powder
- 1/2 tsp Italian seasoning
- 1 tsp salt
- 1/2 tsp pepper

DIRECTIONS:

1. Preheat the oven to 400 degrees F. In a large bowl, add the baby potatoes, broccoli florets, onions, small mushrooms, and baby carrots.
2. Add in the olive oil, salt, pepper, garlic powder and Italian seasoning and toss to evenly coat. Spread the vegetables onto a sheet pan in one even layer.
3. Arrange the sausage slices on the pan over the vegetables. Bake for 30 minutes – make sure to sake halfway through to prevent sticking. Allow to cool.
4. Distribute the Italian sausages and vegetables among the containers and store in the fridge for 2-3 days

NUTRITION: Calories: 321 Fat: 16g Carbs: 23g Protein: 22g

SOUPS

6. Lemon and Egg Pasta Soup

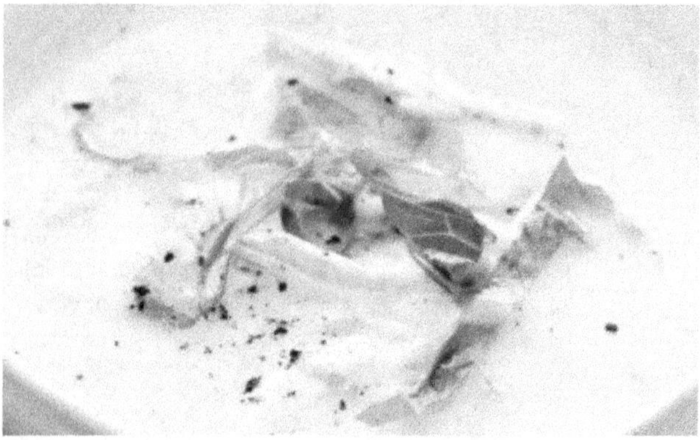

Preparation Time: 15 minutes

Cooking Time: 0 minutes

Servings: 2

INGREDIENTS

- 4 ounces ditalini pasta
- 4 cups fat-free and low-sodium chicken broth
- 2 large whole eggs
- ½ cup fresh lemon juice
- 4 tablespoons chopped fresh parsley
- 1 lemon, thinly sliced for garnish
- Salt and freshly ground pepper to taste

DIRECTIONS

1. Place medium saucepan on medium-high heat. Add chicken broth to it and bring it to a boil, stirring it a couple of times.
2. Bring down the heat to low and allow the broth to simmer for about 5 minutes. Take the saucepan off the heat.
3. Take a bowl and add the eggs into it. Beat them well, add the lemon juice, and beat the eggs again
4. Use a ladle to transfer a single serving of the chicken broth into the egg bowl. Mix them well and then transfer the entire contents of the bowl into the saucepan.
5. Heat the soup while ensuring that the heat is still at low. Keep an eye out on the eggs because they tend to curdle and you need to prevent that from happening by gently stirring the soup.
6. Add salt and pepper to taste, if preferred.
7. Serve hot and garnish with lemon slices and parsley.

NUTRITION: Calories: 161 Protein: 10 g Fat: 2 g Carbohydrate: 65 g

7. Green Creamy Soup

Preparation Time: 10 minutes

Cooking Time: 30 minutes

Servings: 2

INGREDIENTS

- 5 ounces fresh green beans, thinly sliced
- 8 ounces fresh Brussels sprouts, sliced
- 5 cups low-sodium, fat-free vegetable broth
- 1½ cups frozen peas, defrosted
- 4 tablespoons olive oil
- 1 white onion, chopped
- 1 tablespoon freshly squeezed lemon juice
- 4 cloves fresh garlic, minced
- 1 large leek, slice both white parts and sliced green parts thinly but keep them separate
- 1 teaspoon ground coriander
- 1 cup low-fat milk
- Salt and freshly ground pepper to taste
- Croutons for garnish

DIRECTIONS

1. Take out a large skillet and place it over low heat. Add the olive oil and allow the oil to heat up slightly.
2. Add onion and garlic. Cook them until they turn fragrant and soft. Make sure that you do not allow them to turn brown.
3. Add the green parts of the Brussels sprouts, leek, and green beans to the skillet. Add the broth and mix the ingredients well. Bring the broth to a boil. When it starts boiling, lower the heat and let simmer for about 12 minutes.
4. Add lemon juice, peas, and coriander. Let the broth continue to simmer for another 10 minutes, or until the vegetables become tender.
5. Remove the broth mixture from heat and allow it to cool slightly. Transfer the mixture to a blender and pulse until they turn smooth.
6. Take out a saucepan and add the white parts of leek. Add the blended mixture into the saucepan. Place the saucepan over medium high heat and allow the soup to boil. Reduce the heat to low and allow the soup to simmer for about 5 minutes
7. Take out another bowl and add flour and milk. Whisk them until they turn smooth.
8. Add salt and pepper to taste, if preferred.

NUTRITION: Calories: 163 calories Protein: 4 g Fat: 8 g Carbohydrate: 15 g

8. Orzo and Lemon Chicken Soup

Preparation Time: 10 minutes

Cooking Time: 40 minutes

Servings: 2

INGREDIENTS

- 12 ounces skinless, boneless chicken breasts
- 1 tablespoon olive oil
- ½ cup chopped celery
- ½ cup chopped white onion
- 6 cups low-sodium, fat-free chicken broth
- ½ cup sliced carrot
- ½ cup orzo
- ¼ cup chopped fresh dill
- Salt and freshly ground pepper to taste
- Lemon halves

DIRECTIONS

1. Take out a large pot and place it over medium heat. Add olive oil to it and allow it to heat.
2. Add celery and onion. Cook them until the onions are fragrant and the celery is soft.
3. Add chicken, chicken broth, and carrot to the mixture. Add salt and pepper to taste, if preferred.

4. Increase the temperature to medium high heat and allow the broth to boil. When it starts boiling, reduce heat and allow the soup to simmer for about 20 minutes, or until the chicken is cooked.
5. Take out the chicken from the pot, transfer it to a bowl and allow it to cool. Cover the pot so that the ingredients inside are simmering. When the chicken is sufficiently cool, shred the chicken into small pieces.
6. Open the cover of the pot and add orzo. Increase the heat to medium high and allow the broth to boil for about 8 minutes. Make sure that the cover is back on the pot during the boiling process.
7. Remove pot from heat and add dill and the shredded chicken broth.
8. Squeeze lemon juice into the broth. Serve immediately.

NUTRITION: Calories: 248 calories Protein: 25 g Fat: 4 g Carbohydrate: 23 g

9. Chilled Avocado Soup

Preparation Time: 50 minutes

Cooking Time: 0 minutes

Servings: 2

INGREDIENTS

- 3 medium ripe avocados, halved, seeded, peeled, and cut to chunks
- 2 cloves fresh garlic, minced
- 2 cups low-sodium, fat-free chicken broth, divided
- ½ cucumber, peeled and chopped
- ½ cup chopped white onion
- ¼ cup finely diced carrot
- Thin avocado slices for garnish
- Paprika to sprinkle
- Salt and freshly ground pepper to taste
- Hot red pepper sauce to taste

DIRECTIONS

1. Place 6 bowls into the freezer and allow them to chill for half an hour.
2. In the meantime, take out your blender and add garlic, cucumber, avocados, onion, carrot, and 1 cup

broth. Blend all the ingredients together until they turn smooth.

3. Add the remaining broth. Add the salt and pepper and hot sauce to taste, if preferred.
4. Blend all the ingredients again until they are smooth.
5. Take out the chilled bowls and pour the blended ingredients into them.
6. This time, place the bowls in the refrigerator for another 1 hour.
7. When you are ready to serve, top the soup with paprika and slices of avocado.
8. Serve chilled.

NUTRITION: Calories: 255 calories Protein: 4 g Fat: 22 g Carbohydrate: 15 g

10. Broccoli and Potato Soup

Preparation Time: 10 minutes

Cooking Time: 25 minutes

Servings: 2

INGREDIENTS

- 2 cups escarole leaves, rinsed and drained
- 3 tablespoons all-purpose flour
- 3 cups fresh broccoli florets
- 3 scallions, sliced
- 2 cups smoked Gouda cheese, shredded and more for garnish
- 2 cups low-sodium, fat-free chicken broth
- 1 cup almond milk
- 3 medium red-gold potatoes, chopped
- 2 cloves fresh garlic, minced
- Salt and freshly ground pepper to taste

DIRECTIONS

1. Take out a large pot and place it over medium high heat. Add potatoes, garlic, and chicken broth. Bring the mixture to a boil and reduce the heat to low. Allow the mixture to simmer for a while until you notice the potatoes begin to soften

2. Use a fork and mash the potatoes slightly.
3. Add broccoli, milk, and scallions. Continue to heat to a simmer until broccoli turns tender and crispy.
4. Bring down the heat to low and then add the Gouda cheese. Continue stirring until the sauce thickens and the cheese melts.
5. Add salt and pepper for seasoning, if preferred. Serve the soup in 4 equal portions.
6. Add additional cheese and escarole as toppings.

NUTRITION: Calories: 350 calories Protein: 17 g Fat: 14 g Carbohydrate: 42 g

BEEF, PORK & LAMB

11. Pork and Lentil Soup

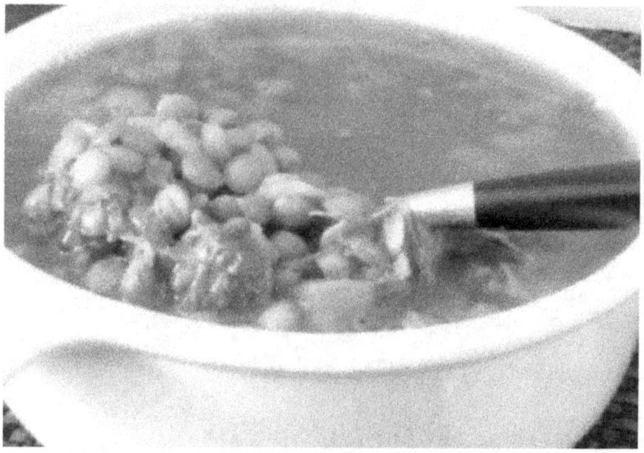

Preparation time: 10 minutes

Cooking time: 1 hour

Servings: 6

INGREDIENTS:

- 1 small yellow onion, chopped
- 1 tablespoon olive oil
- 1 and ½ teaspoons basil, chopped
- 1 and ½ teaspoons ginger, grated
- 3 garlic cloves, chopped
- Salt and black pepper to taste

- ½ teaspoon cumin, ground
- 1 carrot, chopped
- 1-pound pork chops, bone-in 3 ounces brown lentils, rinsed
- 3 cups chicken stock
- 2 tablespoons tomato paste
- 2 tablespoons lime juice
- 1 teaspoon red chili flakes, crushed

DIRECTIONS:

1. Heat a saucepan with the oil over medium heat, add garlic, onion, basil, ginger, salt, pepper and cumin, stir well and cook for 6 minutes.
2. Add carrots, stir and cook 5 more minutes. Add pork and brown for a few minutes. Add lentils, tomato paste and stock, stir, bring to a boil, cover pan and simmer for 50 minutes.
3. Transfer pork to a plate, discard bones, shred it and return to pan. Add chili flakes and lime juice, stir, ladle into bowls and serve.

NUTRITION: Calories 343 Fat 31g Carbs 21g Protein 23g

12. Simple Braised Pork

Preparation time: 40 minutes

Cooking time: 1 hour

Servings: 4

INGREDIENTS:

- 2 pounds pork loin roast, boneless and cubed
- 5 tablespoons butter
- Salt and black pepper to taste
- 2 cups chicken stock
- ½ cup dry white wine
- 2 garlic cloves, minced
- 1 teaspoon thyme, chopped
- 1 thyme spring
- 1 bay leaf
- ½ yellow onion, chopped
- 2 tablespoons white flour
- ¾ pound pearl onions
- ½ pound red grapes

DIRECTIONS:

1. Heat a pan with 2 tablespoons butter over high heat, add pork loin, some salt and pepper, stir, brown for 10 minutes and transfer to a plate.

2. Add wine to the pan, bring to a boil over high heat and cook for 3 minutes.
3. Add stock, garlic, thyme spring, bay leaf, yellow onion and return meat to the pan, bring to a boil, cover, reduce heat to low, cook for 1 hour, strain liquid into another saucepan and transfer pork to a plate.
4. Put pearl onions in a small saucepan, add water to cover, bring to a boil over medium high heat, boil them for 5 minutes, drain, peel them and leave aside for now.
5. In a bowl, mix 2 tablespoons butter with flour and stir well. Add ½ cup of strained cooking liquid and whisk well.
6. Pour this into cooking liquid, bring to a simmer over medium heat and cook for 5 minutes. Add salt and pepper, chopped thyme, pork and pearl onions, cover and simmer for a few minutes.
7. Meanwhile, heat a pan with 1 tablespoon butter, add grapes, stir and cook them for 1-2 minutes. Divide pork meat on plates, drizzle the sauce all over and serve with onions and grapes on the side.

NUTRITION: Calories 320 Fat 31g Carbs 21g Protein 23g

13. Mediterranean Grilled Pork Chops

Preparation time: 1 day & 15 minutes

Cooking time: 20 minutes

Servings: 6

INGREDIENTS:

- 2 pork chops
- ¼ cup olive oil
- 2 yellow onions, sliced
- 2 garlic cloves, minced
- 2 teaspoons mustard
- 1 teaspoon sweet paprika
- Salt and black pepper to taste
- ½ teaspoon oregano, dried
- ½ teaspoon thyme, dried
- A pinch of cayenne pepper

DIRECTIONS:

1. In a small bowl, mix oil with garlic, mustard, paprika, black pepper, oregano, thyme and cayenne and whisk well.

2. In a bowl, combine onions with meat and mustard mix, toss to coat, cover and keep in the fridge for 1 day.
3. Place meat on preheated grill pan over medium high heat, season with salt and cook for 10 minutes on each side.
4. Meanwhile, heat a pan over medium heat, add marinated onions, stir and sauté for 4 minutes. Divide pork chops on plates, add sautéed onions on top and serve.

NUTRITION: Calories 234 Fat 3g Carbs 21g Protein 23g

14. Slow Cooker Mediterranean Beef Roast

Preparation Time: 10 minutes

Cooking Time: 10 hours and 10 minutes

Servings: 2

INGREDIENTS:

- 3 pounds Chuck roast, boneless
- 2 teaspoons Rosemary
- ½ cup Tomatoes, sun-dried and chopped
- 10 cloves Grated garlic
- ½ cup Beef stock
- 2 tablespoons Balsamic vinegar
- ¼ cup Chopped Italian parsley, fresh
- ¼ cup Chopped olives
- 1 teaspoon Lemon zest
- ¼ cup Cheese grits

DIRECTIONS:

1. In the slow cooker, put garlic, sun dried tomatoes, and the beef roast. Add beef stock and Rosemary. Close the cooker and slow cook for 10 hours.

2. After cooking is over, remove the beef, and shred the meet. Discard the fat. Add back the shredded meat to the slow cooker and simmer for 10 minutes.
3. In a small bowl combine lemon zest, parsley, and olives. Cool the mixture until you are ready to serve. Garnish using the refrigerated mix.
4. Serve it over pasta or egg noodles. Top it with cheese grits.

NUTRITION: 314 Calories 19g Fat 1g Carbohydrate 32g Protein 778mg Sodium

15. Slow Cooker Mediterranean Beef Hoagies

Preparation Time: 10 minutes

Cooking Time: 13 hours

Servings: 2

INGREDIENTS:

- 3 pounds Beef top round roast fatless
- ½ teaspoon Onion powder
- ½ teaspoon Black pepper
- 3 cups Low sodium beef broth
- 4 teaspoons Salad dressing mix
- 1 Bay leaf
- 1 tablespoon Garlic, minced
- 2 Red bell peppers, thin strips cut
- 16 ounces Pepperoncino
- 8 slices Sargento Provolone, thin
- 2 ounces Gluten-free bread
- ½ teaspoon salt
- For seasoning:
- 1½ tablespoon Onion powder
- 1½ tablespoon Garlic powder
- 2 tablespoon Dried parsley
- 1 tablespoon stevia

- ½ teaspoon Dried thyme
- 1 tablespoon Dried oregano
- 2 tablespoons Black pepper
- 1 tablespoon Salt
- 6 Cheese slices

DIRECTIONS:

1. Dry the roast with a paper towel. Combine black pepper, onion powder and salt in a small bowl and rub the mixture over the roast.
2. Place the seasoned roast into a slow cooker.
3. Add broth, salad dressing mix, bay leaf, and garlic to the slow cooker. Combine it gently. Close and set to low cooking for 12 hours. After cooking, remove the bay leaf.
4. Take out the cooked beef and shred the beef meet. Put back the shredded beef and add bell peppers and. Add bell peppers and pepperoncino into the slow cooker.
5. Cover the cooker and low cook for 1 hour. Before serving, top each of the bread with 3 ounces of the meat mixture. Top it with a cheese slice. The liquid gravy can be used as a dip.

NUTRITION: 442 Calories 11.5g Fat 37g Carbohydrates 49g Protein 735mg Sodium

16. Beef & Bulgur Meatballs

Preparation Time: 20 minutes

Cooking Time: 28 minutes

Servings: 2

INGREDIENTS:

- ¾ cup uncooked bulgur
- 1-pound ground beef
- ¼ cup shallots, minced
- ¼ cup fresh parsley, minced
- ½ teaspoon ground allspice
- ½ teaspoon ground cumin
- ½ teaspoon ground cinnamon
- ¼ teaspoon red pepper flakes, crushed
- Salt, as required
- 1 tablespoon olive oil

DIRECTIONS:

1. In a large bowl of the cold water, soak the bulgur for about 30 minutes. Drain the bulgur well and then, squeeze with your hands to remove the excess water.
2. In a food processor, add the bulgur, beef, shallot, parsley, spices, salt, and pulse until a smooth mixture is formed.

3. Situate the mixture into a bowl and refrigerate, covered for about 30 minutes. Remove from the refrigerator and make equal sized balls from the beef mixture.
4. In a large nonstick skillet, heat the oil over medium-high heat and cook the meatballs in 2 batches for about 13-14 minutes, flipping frequently. Serve warm.

NUTRITION: 228 Calories 7.4g Fat 0.1g Carbohydrates 3.5g Protein 766mg Sodium

17. Tasty Beef and Broccoli

Preparation Time: 10 minutes

Cooking Time: 15 minutes

Servings: 2

INGREDIENTS:

- 1 and ½ lbs. Flanks steak
- 1 tbsp. Olive oil
- 1 tbsp. Tamari sauce
- 1 cup beef stock
- 1-pound broccoli, florets separated

DIRECTIONS:

1. Combine steak strips with oil and tamari, toss and set aside for 10 minutes. Select your instant pot on sauté mode, place beef strips and brown them for 4 minutes on each side.
2. Stir in stock, cover the pot again and cook on high for 8 minutes. Stir in broccoli, cover and cook on high for 4 minutes more.
3. Portion everything between plates and serve. Enjoy!

NUTRITION: 312 Calories 5g Fat 20g Carbohydrates 4g Protein 694mg Sodium

18. Soy Sauce Beef Roast

Preparation Time: 8 minutes

Cooking Time: 35 minutes

Servings: 2

INGREDIENTS:

- ½ teaspoon beef bouillon
- 1 ½ teaspoon rosemary
- ½ teaspoon minced garlic
- 2 pounds roast beef
- 1/3 cup soy sauce

DIRECTIONS:

1. Combine the soy sauce, bouillon, rosemary, and garlic together in a mixing bowl.
2. Turn on your instant pot. Place the roast, and pour enough water to cover the roast; gently stir to mix well. Seal it tight.
3. Click "MEAT/STEW" Cooking function; set pressure level to "HIGH" and set the Cooking time to 35 minutes. Let the pressure to build to cook the ingredients. Once done, click "CANCEL" setting then click "NPR" Cooking function to release the pressure naturally.

4. Gradually open the lid, and shred the meat. Mix in the shredded meat back in the potting mix and stir well. Transfer in serving containers. Serve warm.

NUTRITION: 423 Calories 14g Fat 12g Carbohydrates 21g Protein 884mg Sodium

19. Slow Cooker Meatloaf

Preparation Time: 10 minutes

Cooking Time: 6 hours and 10 minutes

Servings: 2

INGREDIENTS:

- 2 pounds Ground bison
- 1 Grated zucchini
- 2 large Eggs
- Olive oil cooking spray as required
- 1 Zucchini, shredded
- ½ cup Parsley, fresh, finely chopped
- ½ cup Parmesan cheese, shredded
- 3 tablespoons Balsamic vinegar
- 4 Garlic cloves, grated
- 2 tablespoons Onion minced
- 1 tablespoon Dried oregano
- ½ teaspoon Ground black pepper
- ½ teaspoon Kosher salt
- For the topping:
- ¼ cup Shredded Mozzarella cheese
- ¼ cup Ketchup without sugar
- ¼ cup Freshly chopped parsley

DIRECTIONS:

1. Stripe line the inside of a six-quart slow cooker with aluminum foil. Spray non-stick cooking oil over it.
2. In a large bowl combine ground bison or extra lean ground sirloin, zucchini, eggs, parsley, balsamic vinegar, garlic, dried oregano, sea or kosher salt, minced dry onion, and ground black pepper.
3. Situate this mixture into the slow cooker and form an oblong shaped loaf. Cover the cooker, set on a low heat and cook for 6 hours. After cooking, open the cooker and spread ketchup all over the meatloaf.
4. Now, place the cheese above the ketchup as a new layer and close the slow cooker. Let the meatloaf sit on these two layers for about 10 minutes or until the cheese starts to melt. Garnish with fresh parsley, and shredded Mozzarella cheese.

NUTRITION: 320 Calories 2g Fat 4g Carbohydrates 26g Protein 681mg Sodium

20. Simple Pork Stir Fry

Preparation time: 10 minutes

Cooking time: 15 minutes

Servings: 4

INGREDIENTS:

- 4 ounces bacon, chopped
- 4 ounces snow peas
- 2 tablespoons butter
- 1-pound pork loin, cut into thin strips
- 2 cups mushrooms, sliced
- ¾ cup white wine
- ½ cup yellow onion, chopped
- 3 tablespoons sour cream
- Salt and white pepper to taste

DIRECTIONS:

1. Put snow peas in a saucepan, add water to cover, add a pinch of salt, bring to a boil over medium heat, cook until they are soft, drain and leave aside.
2. Heat a pan over medium high heat, add bacon, cook for a few minutes, drain grease, transfer to a bowl and leave aside.

3. Heat a pan with 1 tablespoon butter over medium heat, add pork strips, salt and pepper to taste, brown for a few minutes and transfer to a plate as well.
4. Return pan to medium heat, add remaining butter and melt it. Add onions and mushrooms, stir and cook for 4 minutes.
5. Add wine, and simmer until it's reduced. Add cream, peas, pork, salt and pepper to taste, stir, heat up, divide between plates, top with bacon and serve.

NUTRITION: Calories 343 Fat 31g Carbs 21g Protein 23g

POULTRY

21. Classic Chicken Cooking with Tomatoes & Tapenade

Preparation Time: 25 minutes

Cooking Time: 25 minutes

Servings: 2

INGREDIENTS:

- 4-5 oz. Chicken breasts, boneless and skinless
- ¼-tsp salt (divided)
- 3-tbsp fresh basil leaves, chopped (divided)
- 1-tbsp olive oil
- 1½-cups cherry tomatoes, halved
- ¼-cup olive tapenade

DIRECTIONS:

1. Arrange the chicken on a sheet of glassine or waxed paper. Sprinkle half of the salt and a third of the basil evenly over the chicken.
2. Press lightly, and flip over the chicken pieces. Sprinkle the remaining salt and another third of the basil.

Cover the seasoned chicken with another sheet of waxed paper.

3. By using a meat mallet or rolling pin, pound the chicken to a half-inch thickness.
4. Heat the olive oil in a 12-inch skillet placed over medium-high heat. Add the pounded chicken breasts.
5. Cook for 6 minutes on each side until the chicken turns golden brown with no traces of pink in the middle. Transfer the browned chicken breasts in a platter, and cover to keep them warm.
6. In the same skillet, add the olive tapenade and tomatoes. Cook for 3 minutes until the tomatoes just begin to be tender.
7. To serve, pour over the tomato-tapenade mixture over the cooked chicken breasts, and top with the remaining basil.

NUTRITION: Calories: 190, Fats: 7g, Dietary Fiber: 1g, Carbohydrates: 6g, Protein: 26g

22. Grilled Grapes & Chicken Chunks

Preparation Time: 15 minutes

Cooking Time: 30 minutes

Servings: 2

INGREDIENTS:

- 2-cloves garlic, minced
- ¼-cup extra-virgin olive oil
- 1-tbsp rosemary, minced
- 1-tbsp oregano, minced
- 1-tsp lemon zest
- ½-tsp red chili flakes, crushed
- 1-lb. Chicken breast, boneless and skinless
- 1¾-cups green grapes, seedless and rinsed
- ½-tsp salt
- 1-tbsp lemon juice
- 2-tbsp extra-virgin olive oil

DIRECTIONS:

1. Combine and mix all the marinade ingredients in a small mixing bowl. Mix well until fully combined. Set aside.
2. Cut the chicken breast into ¾-inch cubes. Alternately thread the chicken and grapes onto 12 skewers. Place

the skewers in a large baking dish to hold them for marinating.

3. Pour the marinade over the skewers, coating them thoroughly. Marinate for 4 to 24 hours.
4. Remove the skewers from the marinade and allow dripping off any excess oil. Sprinkle over with salt.
5. Grill the chicken and grape skewers for 3 minutes on each side until cooked through.
6. To serve, arrange the skewers on a serving platter and drizzle with lemon juice and olive oil.

NUTRITION: Calories: 230, Fats: 20g, Dietary Fiber: 1g, Carbohydrates: 14g, Protein: 1g

23. Turkish Turkey Mini Meatloaves

Preparation Time: 15 minutes

Cooking Time: 20 minutes

Servings: 2

INGREDIENTS:

- 1-lb. Ground turkey breast
- 1-pc egg
- ¼-cup whole-wheat breadcrumbs, crushed
- ¼-cup feta cheese, plus more for topping
- ¼-cup Kalamata olives, halved
- ¼-cup fresh parsley, chopped
- ¼-cup red onion, minced
- ¼-cup + 2-tbsp hummus (refer to Homemade Hummus recipe)
- 2-cloves garlic, minced
- ½-tsp dried basil
- ¼- tsp. Dried oregano
- Salt & pepper
- ½-pc small cucumber, peeled, seeded, and chopped
- 1-pc large tomato, chopped
- 3-tbsp fresh basil, chopped
- ½-lemon, juice

- 1-tsp extra-virgin olive oil
- Salt & pepper

DIRECTIONS:

1. Preheat your oven to 425 ºf.
2. Line a 5"x9" baking sheet with foil, and spray the surfaces with non-stick grease. Set aside.
3. Except for the ¼-cup hummus, combine and mix all the turkey meatloaf ingredients in a large mixing bowl. Mix well until fully combined.
4. Divide mixture equally into 4 portions. Form the portions into loaves. Spread a tablespoon of the remaining hummus on each meatloaf. Place the loaves on the greased baking sheet.
5. Bake for 20 minutes until the loaves no longer appear pink in the center. (Ensure the meatloaf cooks through by inserting a meat thermometer and the reading reaches 165 ºf.)
6. Combine and mix all the topping ingredients in a small mixing bowl. Mix well until fully combined.
7. To serve, spoon the topping over the cooked meatloaves.

NUTRITION: Calories: 130, Fats: 7g, Dietary Fiber: 4g, Carbohydrates: 14g, Protein: 6g

24. Charred Chicken Souvlaki Skewers

Preparation Time: 20 minutes

Cooking Time: 15 minutes

Servings: 2

INGREDIENTS:

- ½-cup olive oil
- ½-cup fresh squeezed lemon juice
- 1-tbsp red wine vinegar
- 1-tbsp finely minced garlic (or garlic puree from a jar)
- 1-tbsp dried Greek oregano
- 1-tsp dried thyme
- 6-pcs chicken breasts, boneless, skinless, with trimmed off tendons and fats
- Fresh cucumber and cherry tomatoes for garnish

DIRECTIONS:

1. Combine and mix all the marinade ingredients in a small mixing bowl. Mix well until fully combined.
2. Slice each chicken breast crosswise into six 1-inch strips.
3. Place the chicken strips into a large plastic container with a tight-fitting lid.

4. Pour the marinade into the plastic container, and seal with its lid. Gently shake the container and turn it over so that the marinade evenly coats all of the meat. Refrigerate the sealed plastic container to marinate for 8 hours or more.
5. Spray the grill's surfaces with non-stick grease. Preheat your charcoal or gas barbecue grill to medium-high heat.
6. Take the chicken out and let it cool to room temperature. Drain the chicken pieces and thread them onto skewers. (Try to thread six pieces for each skewer and fold over each chicken piece so it will not spin around the skewer.)
7. Grill the chicken souvlaki skewers for 15 minutes, turning once after seeing the appearance of desirable grill marks.
8. To serve, place the souvlaki on a serving plate alongside the cucumber and tomato garnish.

NUTRITION: Calories: 360, Fats: 26g, Dietary Fiber: 0g, Carbohydrates: 3g, Protein: 30g

25. Lemon Caper Chicken

Preparation Time: 10 minutes

Cooking Time: 15 minutes

Servings: 2

INGREDIENTS:

- 2 tablespoon virgin olive oil
- 2 chicken breasts (boneless, skinless, cut in half, pound to ¾ an inch thick)
- ¼ cup capers
- 2 lemons (wedges)
- 1 teaspoon oregano
- 1 teaspoon basil
- ½ teaspoon black pepper

DIRECTIONS:

1. Take a large skillet and place it on your stove and add the olive oil to it. Turn the heat to medium and allow it to warm up.
2. As the oil heats up season your chicken breast with the oregano, basil, and black pepper on each side.
3. Place your chicken breast into the hot skillet and cook on each side for five minutes.

4. Transfer the chicken from the skillet to your dinner plate. Top with capers and serve with a few lemon wedges.

NUTRITION: Calories – 182, Carbs - 3.4 g, Protein - 26.6 g, Fat - 8.2 g

26. Herb Roasted Chicken

Preparation Time: 20 minutes

Cooking Time: 45 minutes

Servings: 2

INGREDIENTS:

- 1 tablespoon virgin olive oil
- 1 whole chicken
- 2 rosemary springs
- 3 garlic cloves (peeled)
- 1 lemon (cut in half)
- 1 teaspoon sea salt
- 1 teaspoon black pepper

DIRECTIONS:

1. Turn your oven to 450 degrees F.
2. Take your whole chicken and pat it dry using paper towels. Then rub in the olive oil. Remove the leaves from one of the springs of rosemary and scatter them over the chicken. Sprinkle the sea salt and black pepper over top. Place the other whole sprig of rosemary into the cavity of the chicken. Then add in the garlic cloves and lemon halves.

3. Place the chicken into a roasting pan and then place it into the oven. Allow the chicken to bake for 1 hour, then check that the internal temperature should be at least 165 degrees F. If the chicken begins to brown too much, cover it with foil and return it to the oven to finish cooking.
4. When the chicken has cooked to the appropriate temperature remove it from the oven. Let it rest for at least 20 minutes before carving.
5. Serve with a large side of roasted or steamed vegetables or your favorite salad.

NUTRITION: Calories – 309, Carbs - 1.5 g, Protein - 27.2 g, Fat - 21.3 g

27. Italian Chicken Meatballs

Preparation Time: 20 minutes

Cooking Time: 32 minutes

Servings: 20

INGREDIENTS:

- 3 tomatoes
- Kosher salt
- ½ cup of freshly chopped parsley
- 1 teaspoon of dry oregano
- Kosher salt
- ½ teaspoon of fresh thyme
- ¼ teaspoon of sweet paprika
- 1 red onion
- 1 lb. Of ground chicken
- ½ minced garlic cloves
- Black pepper
- 1 raw egg
- ¼ cup of freshly grated parmesan cheese
- Extra virgin olive oil.

DIRECTIONS:

1. Heat the oven to 375 degrees and get a cooking pan. Coat with extra virgin olive oil and set aside.

2. Get a large bowl and mix your tomatoes with kosher salt and thinly chopped onions.
3. Add half of your fresh thyme and sprinkle a little extra virgin olive oil on it again.
4. Transfer this to your cooking and use a spoon to spread. Add ground chicken to the mixing bowl you recently used, and add egg, parmesan cheese and oregano.
5. Include paprika, garlic, the other half of thyme, chopped parsley and black pepper.
6. Sprinkle a little amount of extra virgin olive oil on it, and mix till the meatball mixture is combined. Form about 1 ½ inch chicken meatballs with the mixture and cut it all to this size.
7. Get another cooking pan and arrange these meatballs in it. Add tomatoes and onions, and blend them with the meatballs. Bake in your preheated oven for about 30 min.
8. Your meatballs should turn golden brown, you can make them more colorful by removing them and coating them with extra virgin olive oil before you continue baking.
9. But that is not necessary. A couple of minutes after this, your meatballs cam is served.
10. No surprises, your tomatoes are fast falling.

NUTRITION: 79 kcal, 74.7mg of sodium, 1.4g of sugar, 301.1g of potassium, 0.92g of fiber, 44.2mg of calcium, 0.94g of iron, 4.1g of carbs, 7.8g of protein.

28. Oven Roasted Garlic Chicken Thigh

Preparation time: 10 minutes

Cooking time: 55 minutes

Servings: 2

INGREDIENTS:

- 8 chicken thighs
- Salt and pepper as needed
- 1 tablespoon extra-virgin olive oil
- 6 cloves garlic, peeled and crushed
- 1 jar (10 ounces) roasted red peppers, drained and chopped
- 1 1/2 pounds potatoes, diced
- 2 cups cherry tomatoes, halved
- 1/3 cup capers, sliced
- 1 teaspoon dried Italian seasoning
- 1 tablespoon fresh basil

DIRECTIONS:

1. Season chicken with kosher salt and black pepper.
2. Take a cast-iron skillet over medium-high heat and heat up olive oil.
3. Sear the chicken on both sides.

4. Add remaining ingredients except for basil and stir well.
5. Remove heat and place cast iron skillet in the oven.
6. Bake for 45 minutes at 400 degrees Fahrenheit until the internal temperature reaches 165 degrees Fahrenheit.
7. Serve and enjoy!

NUTRITION: Calories: 500, Fat: 23g, Carbs: 37g, Protein: 35g

29. Mediterranean bowl

Preparation Time: 25 minutes

Cooking Time: 30 minutes

Servings: 2

INGREDIENTS:

- 2 chicken breasts (chopped into 4 halves)
- 2 diced onions
- 2 bottles of lemon pepper marinade
- 2 diced green bell pepper
- 4 lemon juices
- 8 cloves of crushed garlic.
- 5 teaspoon of olive oil
- Feta cheese
- 1 grape tomato
- 1 large-sized diced zucchini and 1 small-sized. Otherwise, use two medium-sized diced zucchinis.
- Salt and pepper (according to your desired taste), 4 cups of water.
- Kalamata olives (as much as you fancy)
- 1 cup of garbanzo beans

NUTRITION: 541 Cal, 34g of protein, 1423mg of potassium, 12g of fiber, 15g of sugar, 72mg of cholesterol, 4g of fat, 45g of carbs.

30. Grilled Chicken Breasts

Preparation Time: 10 minutes

Cooking Time: 15 minutes

Servings: 2

INGREDIENTS:

- Boneless skinless chicken breast, 4.
- Lemon juice, 3 tbsp.
- Olive oil, 3 tbsp.
- Chopped fresh parsley, 3 tbsp.
- Minced garlic cloves, 3.
- Paprika, 1 tsp.
- Dried oregano, ½ tsp.
- Salt and pepper, to taste.

DIRECTIONS:

1. In a large Ziploc bag, mix well oregano, paprika, garlic, parsley, olive oil, and lemon juice.
2. Pierce chicken with a knife several times and sprinkle with salt and pepper.
3. Add chicken to bag and marinate 20 minutes or up to two days in the fridge.
4. Remove chicken from bag and grill for 5 minutes per side in a 3500 F preheated grill.

5. When cooked, transfer to a plate for 5 minutes before slicing.
6. Serve and enjoy with a side of rice or salad

NUTRITION: Calories: 238, Protein: 24 g, Carbohydrates: 2 g, Fats: 19 g

FISH & SEAFOOD

31. Fast Seafood Paella

Preparation time: 15 minutes

Cooking time: 20 minutes

Servings: 4

INGREDIENTS:

- ¼ cup plus 1 tablespoon extra-virgin olive oil
- 1 large onion, finely chopped
- 2 tomatoes, peeled and chopped
- 1½ tablespoons garlic powder
- 1½ cups medium-grain Spanish paella rice or arborio rice
- 2 carrots, finely diced
- Salt, to taste
- 1 tablespoon sweet paprika
- 8 ounces (227 g) lobster meat or canned crab
- ½ cup frozen peas
- 3 cups chicken stock, plus more if needed
- 1 cup dry white wine
- 6 jumbo shrimp, unpeeled

- $^{1}/_{3}$ pound (136 g) calamari rings
- 1 lemon, halved

DIRECTIONS:

1. In a large sauté pan or skillet (16-inch is ideal), heat the oil over medium heat until small bubbles start to escape from oil.
2. Add the onion and cook for about 3 minutes, until fragrant, then add tomatoes and garlic powder. Cook for 5 to 10 minutes, until the tomatoes are reduced by half and the consistency is sticky.
3. Stir in the rice, carrots, salt, paprika, lobster, and peas and mix well. In a pot or microwave-safe bowl, heat the chicken stock to almost boiling, then add it to the rice mixture. Bring to a simmer, then add the wine.
4. Smooth out the rice in the bottom of the pan. Cover and cook on low for 10 minutes, mixing occasionally, to prevent burning.
5. Top the rice with the shrimp, cover, and cook for 5 more minutes. Add additional broth to the pan if the rice looks dried out.
6. Right before removing the skillet from the heat, add the calamari rings. Toss the ingredients frequently.
7. In about 2 minutes, the rings will look opaque. Remove the pan from the heat immediately—you

don't want the paella to overcook). Squeeze fresh lemon juice over the dish.

NUTRITION: Calories: 632 Fat: 20g Protein: 34g Carbs: 71g

32. Crispy Fried Sardines

Preparation time: 15 minutes

Cooking time: 5 minutes

Servings: 4

INGREDIENTS:

- Avocado oil, as needed
- 1½ pounds (680 g) whole fresh sardines, scales removed
- 1 teaspoon salt
- 1 teaspoon freshly ground black pepper
- 2 cups flour

DIRECTIONS:

1. Preheat a deep skillet over medium heat. Pour in enough oil so there is about 1 inch of it in the pan. Season the fish with the salt and pepper.
2. Dredge the fish in the flour so it is completely covered. Slowly drop in 1 fish at a time, making sure not to overcrowd the pan.
3. Cook for about 3 minutes on each side or just until the fish begins to brown on all sides. Serve warm.

NUTRITION: Calories: 794 Fat: 47g Protein: 48g Carbs: 44g

33. Orange Roasted Salmon

Preparation time: 15 minutes

Cooking time: 25 minutes

Servings: 4

INGREDIENTS:

- ½ cup extra-virgin olive oil, divided
- 2 tablespoons balsamic vinegar
- 2 tablespoons garlic powder, divided
- 1 tablespoon cumin seeds
- 1 teaspoon sea salt, divided
- 1 teaspoon freshly ground black pepper, divided
- 2 teaspoons smoked paprika
- 4 (8-ounce / 227-g) salmon fillets, skinless
- 2 small red onion, thinly sliced
- ½ cup halved Campari tomatoes
- 1 small fennel bulb, thinly sliced lengthwise
- 1 large carrot, thinly sliced
- 8 medium portobello mushrooms
- 8 medium radishes, sliced ⅛ inch thick
- ½ cup dry white wine
- ½ lime, zested
- Handful cilantro leaves
- ½ cup halved pitted Kalamata olives

- 1 orange, thinly sliced
- 4 roasted sweet potatoes, cut in wedges lengthwise

DIRECTIONS:

1. Preheat the oven to 375°f (190°c). In a medium bowl, mix 6 tablespoons of olive oil, the balsamic vinegar, 1 tablespoon of garlic powder, the cumin seeds, ¼ teaspoon of sea salt, ¼ teaspoon of pepper, and the paprika.
2. Put the salmon in the bowl and marinate while preparing the vegetables, about 10 minutes.
3. Heat an oven-safe sauté pan or skillet on medium-high heat and sear the top of the salmon for about 2 minutes, or until lightly brown. Set aside.
4. Add the remaining 2 tablespoons of olive oil to the same skillet. Once it's hot, add the onion, tomatoes, fennel, carrot, mushrooms, radishes, the remaining 1 teaspoon of garlic powder, ¾ teaspoon of salt, and ¾ teaspoon of pepper.
5. Mix well and cook for 5 to 7 minutes, until fragrant. Add wine and mix well. Place the salmon on top of the vegetable mixture, browned-side up.
6. Sprinkle the fish with lime zest and cilantro and place the olives around the fish. Put orange slices over the fish and cook for about 7 additional minutes.
7. While this is baking, add the sliced sweet potato wedges on a baking sheet and bake this alongside the

skillet. Remove from the oven, cover the skillet tightly, and let rest for about 3 minutes.

NUTRITION: Calories: 841 Fat: 41g Protein: 59g Carbs: 60g

34. Lemon Rosemary Branzino

Preparation time: 15 minutes

Cooking time: 30 minutes

Servings: 4

INGREDIENTS:

- 4 tablespoons extra-virgin olive oil, divided
- 2 (8-ounce / 227-g) branzino fillets, preferably at least 1 inch thick
- 1 garlic clove, minced
- 1 bunch scallions, white part only, thinly sliced
- ½ cup sliced pitted Kalamata or other good-quality black olives
- 1 large carrot, cut into ¼-inch rounds
- 10 to 12 small cherry tomatoes, halved
- ½ cup dry white wine
- 2 tablespoons paprika
- 2 teaspoons kosher salt
- ½ tablespoon ground chili pepper, preferably Turkish or Aleppo
- 2 rosemary sprigs or 1 tablespoon dried rosemary
- 1 small lemon, very thinly sliced

DIRECTIONS:

1. Warm a large, oven-safe sauté pan or skillet over high heat until hot, about 2 minutes. Carefully add 1 tablespoon of olive oil and heat until it shimmers, 10 to 15 seconds.
2. Brown the branzino fillets for 2 minutes, skin-side up. Carefully flip the fillets skin-side down and cook for another 2 minutes, until browned. Set aside.
3. Swirl 2 tablespoons of olive oil around the skillet to coat evenly. Add the garlic, scallions, kalamata olives, carrot, and tomatoes, and let the vegetables sauté for 5 minutes, until softened.
4. Add the wine, stirring until all ingredients are well integrated. Carefully place the fish over the sauce. Preheat the oven to 450ºf (235ºc).
5. While the oven is heating, brush the fillets with 1 tablespoon of olive oil and season with paprika, salt, and chili pepper.
6. Top each fillet with a rosemary sprig and several slices of lemon. Scatter the olives over fish and around the pan. Roast until lemon slices are browned or singed, about 10 minutes.

NUTRITION: calories: 725 fat: 43g protein: 58g carbs: 25g

35. Almond-Crusted Swordfish

Preparation time: 15 minutes

Cooking time: 15 minutes

Servings: 4

INGREDIENTS:

- ½ cup almond flour
- ¼ cup crushed Marcona almonds
- ½ to 1 teaspoon salt, divided
- 2 pounds (907 g) Swordfish, preferably 1 inch thick
- 1 large egg, beaten (optional)
- ¼ cup pure apple cider
- ¼ cup extra-virgin olive oil, plus more for frying
- 3 to 4 sprigs flat-leaf parsley, chopped
- 1 lemon, juiced
- 1 tablespoon Spanish paprika
- 5 medium baby portobello mushrooms, chopped (optional)
- 4 or 5 chopped scallions, both green and white parts
- 3 to 4 garlic cloves, peeled
- ¼ cup chopped pitted Kalamata olives

DIRECTIONS:

1. On a dinner plate, spread the flour and crushed Marcona almonds and mix in the salt. Alternately, pour the flour, almonds, and ¼ teaspoon of salt into a large plastic food storage bag.
2. Add the fish and coat it with the flour mixture. If a thicker coat is desired, repeat this step after dipping the fish in the egg (if using).
3. In a measuring cup, combine the apple cider, ¼ cup of olive oil, parsley, lemon juice, paprika, and ¼ teaspoon of salt. Mix well and set aside.
4. In a large, heavy-bottom sauté pan or skillet, pour the olive oil to a depth of ⅛ inch and heat on medium heat.
5. Once the oil is hot, add the fish and brown for 3 to 5 minutes, then turn the fish over and add the mushrooms (If using), scallions, garlic, and olives.
6. Cook for an additional 3 minutes. Once the other side of the fish is brown, remove the fish from the pan and set aside.
7. Pour the cider mixture into the skillet and mix well with the vegetables. Put the fried fish into the skillet on top of the mixture and cook with sauce on medium-low heat for 10 minutes, until the fish flakes easily with a fork.

8. Carefully remove the fish from the pan and plate. Spoon the sauce over the fish. Serve with white rice or home-fried potatoes.

NUTRITION: Calories: 620 Fat: 37g Protein: 63g Carbs: 10g

36. Sea Bass Crusted with Moroccan Spices

Preparation time: 15 minutes

Cooking time: 40 minutes

Servings: 4

INGREDIENTS:

- 1½ teaspoons ground turmeric, divided
- ¾ teaspoon saffron
- ½ teaspoon ground cumin
- ¼ teaspoon kosher salt
- ¼ teaspoon freshly ground black pepper
- 1½ pounds (680 g) sea bass fillets, about ½ inch thick
- 8 tablespoons extra-virgin olive oil, divided
- 8 garlic cloves, divided (4 minced cloves and 4 sliced)
- 6 medium baby portobello mushrooms, chopped
- 1 large carrot, sliced on an angle
- 2 sun-dried tomatoes, thinly sliced (optional)
- 2 tablespoons tomato paste
- 1 (15-ounce / 425-g) can chickpeas, drained and rinsed
- 1½ cups low-sodium vegetable broth
- ¼ cup white wine
- 1 tablespoon ground coriander (optional)

- 1 cup sliced artichoke hearts marinated in olive oil
- ½ cup pitted Kalamata olives
- ½ lemon, juiced
- ½ lemon, cut into thin rounds
- 4 to 5 rosemary sprigs or 2 tablespoons dried rosemary
- Fresh cilantro, for garnish

DIRECTIONS:

1. In a small mixing bowl, combine 1 teaspoon turmeric and the saffron and cumin. Season with salt and pepper. Season both sides of the fish with the spice mixture.
2. Add 3 tablespoons of olive oil and work the fish to make sure it's well coated with the spices and the olive oil.
3. In a large sauté pan or skillet, heat 2 tablespoons of olive oil over medium heat until shimmering but not smoking. Sear the top side of the sea bass for about 1 minute, or until golden. Remove and set aside.
4. In the same skillet, add the minced garlic and cook very briefly, tossing regularly, until fragrant. Add the mushrooms, carrot, sun-dried tomatoes (if using), and tomato paste.
5. Cook for 3 to 4 minutes over medium heat, tossing frequently, until fragrant. Add the chickpeas, broth, wine, coriander (if using), and the sliced garlic.

6. Stir in the remaining ½ teaspoon ground turmeric. Raise the heat, if needed, and bring to a boil, then lower heat to simmer. Cover part of the way and let the sauce simmer for about 20 minutes, until thickened.
7. Carefully add the seared fish to the skillet. Ladle a bit of the sauce on top of the fish. Add the artichokes, olives, lemon juice and slices, and rosemary sprigs.
8. Cook another 10 minutes or until the fish is fully cooked and flaky. Garnish with fresh cilantro.

NUTRITION: Calories: 696 Fat: 41g Protein: 48g Carbs: 37g

37. Cilantro Lemon Shrimp

Preparation time: 20 minutes

Cooking time: 10 minutes

Servings: 4

INGREDIENTS:

- 1/3 cup lemon juice
- 4 garlic cloves
- 1 cup fresh cilantro leaves
- ½ teaspoon ground coriander
- 3 tablespoons extra-virgin olive oil
- 1 teaspoon salt
- 1½ pounds (680 g) large shrimp (21 to 25), deveined and shells removed

DIRECTIONS:

1. In a food processor, pulse the lemon juice, garlic, cilantro, coriander, olive oil, and salt 10 times. Put the shrimp in a bowl or plastic zip-top bag, pour in the cilantro marinade, and let sit for 15 minutes.
2. Preheat a skillet on high heat. Put the shrimp and marinade in the skillet. Cook the shrimp for 3 minutes on each side. Serve warm.

NUTRITION: Calories: 225 Fat: 12g Protein: 28g Carbs: 5g

38. Shrimp with Garlic and Mushrooms

Preparation time: 15 minutes

Cooking time: 15 minutes

Servings: 4

INGREDIENTS:

- 1 pound (454 g) peeled and deveined fresh shrimp
- 1 teaspoon salt
- 1 cup extra-virgin olive oil
- 8 large garlic cloves, thinly sliced
- 4 ounces (113 g) sliced mushrooms (shiitake, baby bella, or button)
- ½ teaspoon red pepper flakes
- ¼ cup chopped fresh flat-leaf Italian parsley
- Zucchini noodles or riced cauliflower, for serving

DIRECTIONS:

1. Rinse the shrimp and pat dry. Place in a small bowl and sprinkle with the salt. In a large rimmed, thick skillet, heat the olive oil over medium-low heat.
2. Add the garlic and heat until very fragrant, 3 to 4 minutes, reducing the heat if the garlic starts to burn.

3. Add the mushrooms and sauté for 5 minutes, until softened. Add the shrimp and red pepper flakes and sauté until the shrimp begins to turn pink, another 3 to 4 minutes.
4. Remove from the heat and stir in the parsley. Serve over zucchini noodles or riced cauliflower.

NUTRITION: Calories: 620 Fat: 56g Protein: 24g Carbs: 4g

39. Pistachio-Crusted Whitefish

Preparation Time: 10 minutes

Cooking Time: 20 minutes

Servings: 2

INGREDIENTS:

- ¼ cup shelled pistachios
- 1 tablespoon fresh parsley
- 1 tablespoon grated Parmesan cheese
- 1 tablespoon panko bread crumbs
- 2 tablespoons olive oil
- ¼ teaspoon salt
- 10 ounces skinless whitefish (1 large piece or 2 smaller ones)

DIRECTIONS:

1. Preheat the oven to 350°F and set the rack to the middle position. Line a sheet pan with foil or parchment paper.
2. Combine all of the ingredients except the fish in a mini food processor, and pulse until the nuts are finely ground.

3. Alternatively, you can mince the nuts with a chef's knife and combine the ingredients by hand in a small bowl.
4. Place the fish on the sheet pan. Spread the nut mixture evenly over the fish and pat it down lightly.
5. Bake the fish for 20 to 30 minutes, depending on the thickness, until it flakes easily with a fork.
6. Keep in mind that a thicker cut of fish takes a bit longer to bake. You'll know it's done when it's opaque, flakes apart easily with a fork, or reaches an internal temperature of 145°F

NUTRITION: Calories – 185, Carbs - 23.8 g, Protein - 10.1 g, Fat - 5.2 g

40. Seafood Risotto

Preparation time: 15 minutes

Cooking time: 30 minutes

Servings: 4

INGREDIENTS:

- 6 cups vegetable broth
- 3 tablespoons extra-virgin olive oil
- 1 large onion, chopped
- 3 cloves garlic, minced
- ½ teaspoon saffron threads
- 1½ cups arborio rice
- 1½ teaspoons salt
- 8 ounces (227 g) shrimp (21 to 25), peeled and deveined
- 8 ounces (227 g) scallops

DIRECTIONS:

1. In a large saucepan over medium heat, bring the broth to a low simmer. In a large skillet over medium heat, cook the olive oil, onion, garlic, and saffron for 3 minutes.

2. Add the rice, salt, and 1 cup of the broth to the skillet. Stir the ingredients together and cook over low heat until most of the liquid is absorbed.
3. Repeat steps with broth, adding ½ cup of broth at a time, and cook until all but ½ cup of the broth is absorbed.
4. Add the shrimp and scallops when you stir in the final ½ cup of broth. Cover and let cook for 10 minutes. Serve warm.

NUTRITION: Calories: 460 Fat: 12g Protein: 24g Carbs: 64g

APPETIZERS & SNACKS

41. Speedy Sweet Potato Chips

Preparation Time: 15 Minutes

Cooking Time: 0 Minutes

Servings: 4

INGREDIENTS:

- 1 large Sweet potato
- 1 tbsp Extra virgin olive oil
- Salt

DIRECTIONS:

1. 300°F preheated oven. Slice your potato into nice, thin slices that resemble fries.
2. Toss the potato slices with salt and extra virgin olive oil in a bowl. Bake for about one hour, flipping every 15 minutes until crispy and browned.

NUTRITION: Calories: 150 Carbs: 16g Fat: 9g Protein: 1g

42. Nachos with Hummus (Mediterranean Inspired)

Preparation Time: 15 Minutes

Cooking Time: 20 Minutes

Servings: 4

INGREDIENTS:

- 4 cups salted pita chips
- 1 (8 oz.) Red pepper (roasted)
- Hummus
- 1 tsp Finely shredded lemon peel
- ¼ cup Chopped pitted Kalamata olives
- ¼ cup crumbled feta cheese
- 1 plum (Roma) tomato, seeded, chopped
- ½ cup chopped cucumber
- 1 tsp Chopped fresh oregano leaves

DIRECTIONS:

1. 400°F preheated oven. Arrange the pita chips on a heatproof platter and drizzle with hummus.
2. Top with olives, tomato, cucumber, and cheese and bake until warmed through. Sprinkle lemon zest and oregano and enjoy while it's hot.

NUTRITION: Calories: 130 Carbs: 18g Fat: 5g Protein: 4g

43. Stuffed Celery

Preparation Time: 15 Minutes

Cooking Time: 20 Minutes

Servings: 3

INGREDIENTS:

- Olive oil
- 1 clove garlic, minced
- 2 tbsp Pine nuts
- 2 tbsp dry-roasted sunflower seeds
- ¼ cup Italian cheese blend, shredded
- 8 stalks celery leaves
- 1 (8-ounce) fat-free cream cheese
- Cooking spray

DIRECTIONS:

1. Sauté garlic and pine nuts over a medium setting for the heat until the nuts are golden brown. Cut off the wide base and tops from celery.
2. Remove two thin strips from the round side of the celery to create a flat surface.
3. Mix Italian cheese and cream cheese in a bowl and spread into cut celery stalks.

4. Sprinkle half of the celery pieces with sunflower seeds and a half with the pine nut mixture. Cover mixture and let stand for at least 4 hours before eating.

NUTRITION: Calories: 64 Carbs: 2g Fat: 6g Protein: 1g

44. Hummus and Olive Pita Bread

Preparation Time: 5 Minutes

Cooking Time: 0 Minutes

Servings: 3

INGREDIENTS:

- 7 pita bread cut into 6 wedges each
- 1 (7 ounces) container plain hummus
- 1 tbsp Greek vinaigrette
- ½ cup Chopped pitted Kalamata olives

DIRECTIONS:

1. Spread the hummus on a serving plate—Mix vinaigrette and olives in a bowl and spoon over the hummus. Enjoy with wedges of pita bread.

NUTRITION: Calories: 225 Carbs: 40g Fat: 5g Protein: 9g

45. Butternut Squash Fries

Preparation Time: 5 Minutes

Cooking Time: 10 Minutes

Servings: 2

INGREDIENTS:

- 1 Butternut squash
- 1 tbsp Extra virgin olive oil
- ½ tbsp Grapeseed oil
- 1/8 tsp Sea salt

DIRECTIONS:

1. Remove seeds from the squash and cut into thin slices. Coat with extra virgin olive oil and grapeseed oil. Add a sprinkle of salt and toss to coat well.
2. Arrange the squash slices onto three baking sheets and bake for 10 minutes until crispy.

NUTRITION: Calories: 40 Carbs: 10g Fat: 0g Protein: 1g

DESSERTS

46. Berry and Rhubarb Cobbler

Preparation time: 15 minutes

Cooking time: 35 minutes

Servings: 8

INGREDIENTS:

- Cobbler:
- 1 cup fresh raspberries
- 2 cups fresh blueberries
- 1 cup sliced (½-inch) rhubarb pieces
- 1 tablespoon arrowroot powder
- ¼ cup unsweetened apple juice
- 2 tablespoons melted coconut oil
- ¼ cup raw honey
- Topping:
- 1 cup almond flour
- 1 tablespoon arrowroot powder
- ½ cup shredded coconut
- ¼ cup raw honey
- ½ cup coconut oil

DIRECTIONS:

1. Preheat the oven to 350°f (180°c). Grease a baking dish with melted coconut oil. Combine the ingredients for the cobbler in a large bowl. Stir to mix well. Spread the mixture in the single layer on the baking dish. Set aside.
2. Combine the almond flour, arrowroot powder, and coconut in a bowl. Stir to mix well. Fold in the honey and coconut oil. Stir with a fork until the mixture crumbled.
3. Spread the topping over the cobbler, then bake in the preheated oven for 35 minutes or until frothy and golden brown. Serve immediately.

NUTRITION: Calories: 305 Fat: 22.1g Protein: 3.2g Carbs: 29.8g

47. Citrus Cranberry and Quinoa Energy Bites

Preparation time: 15 minutes

Cooking time: 0 minutes

Servings: 12 bites

INGREDIENTS:

- 2 tablespoons almond butter
- 2 tablespoons maple syrup
- ¾ cup cooked quinoa
- 1 tablespoon dried cranberries
- 1 tablespoon chia seeds
- ¼ cup ground almonds
- ¼ cup sesame seeds, toasted
- Zest of 1 orange
- ½ teaspoon vanilla extract

DIRECTIONS:

1. Line a baking sheet with parchment paper. Combine the butter and maple syrup in a bowl. Stir to mix well.
2. Fold in the remaining ingredients and stir until the mixture holds together and smooth. Divide the mixture into 12 equal parts, then shape each part into a ball.

3. Arrange the balls on the baking sheet, then refrigerate for at least 15 minutes. Serve chilled.

NUTRITION: Calories: 110 Fat: 10.8g Protein: 3.1g Carbs: 4.9g

48. Chocolate, Almond, and Cherry Clusters

Preparation time: 15 minutes

Cooking time: 3 minutes

Servings: 10 clusters

INGREDIENTS:

- 1 cup dark chocolate (60% cocoa or higher), chopped
- 1 tablespoon coconut oil
- ½ cup dried cherries
- 1 cup roasted salted almonds

DIRECTIONS:

1. Line a baking sheet with parchment paper. Melt the chocolate and coconut oil in a saucepan for 3 minutes. Stir constantly.
2. Turn off the heat and mix in the cherries and almonds. Drop the mixture on the baking sheet with a spoon. Place the sheet in the refrigerator and chill for at least 1 hour or until firm. Serve chilled.

NUTRITION: Calories: 197 Fat: 13.2g Protein: 4.1g Carbs: 17.8g

49. Apple and Berries Ambrosia

Preparation time: 15 minutes

Cooking time: 0 minutes

Servings: 4

INGREDIENTS:

- 2 cups unsweetened coconut milk, chilled
- 2 tablespoons raw honey
- 1 apple, peeled, cored, and chopped
- 2 cups fresh raspberries
- 2 cups fresh blueberries

DIRECTIONS:

1. Spoon the chilled milk in a large bowl, then mix in the honey. Stir to mix well.
2. Then mix in the remaining ingredients. Stir to coat the fruits well and serve immediately.

NUTRITION: Calories: 386 Fat: 21.1g Protein: 4.2g Carbs: 45.9g

50. Chocolate and Avocado Mousse

Preparation time: 15 minutes

Cooking time: 5 minutes

Servings: 4-6

INGREDIENTS:

- 8 ounces (227 g) dark chocolate (60% cocoa or higher), chopped
- ¼ cup unsweetened coconut milk
- 2 tablespoons coconut oil
- 2 ripe avocados, deseeded
- ¼ cup raw honey
- Sea salt, to taste

DIRECTIONS:

1. Put the chocolate in a saucepan. Pour in the coconut milk and add the coconut oil. Cook for 3 minutes or until the chocolate and coconut oil melt. Stir constantly.
2. Put the avocado in a food processor, then drizzle with honey and melted chocolate. Pulse to combine until smooth.
3. Pour the mixture in a serving bowl, then sprinkle with salt. Refrigerate to chill for 30 minutes and serve.

NUTRITION: Calories: 654 Fat: 46.8g Protein: 7.2g Carbs: 55.9g

CPSIA information can be obtained
at www.ICGtesting.com
Printed in the USA
LVHW020745260521
688475LV00014B/1497

9 781803 040080